FLAGYL (Metronidazole)

Guide to treat bacterial, pneumonia and other respiratory tract infections; certain infections of skin, eye, lymphatic, intestinal, genital and urinary systems

Bella Asheville

Table of Contents

Chapter 1

Introduction

Flagyl, also known as metronidazole, is an antibiotic medication that has been used for over 60 years to treat various infections caused by bacteria and parasites. It is a very common and widely-prescribed drug, with over 12 million prescriptions written in the United States each year.

The history of Flagyl dates back to the 1930s when researchers discovered that certain bacteria in the soil produced a substance called nitroimidazole. It wasn't until 1959 that scientists were able to synthesize this compound and create metronidazole, the active ingredient in Flagyl. The drug was initially used to treat trichomoniasis, a sexually transmitted infection caused by a parasite. However, it was soon discovered that it was also effective against certain types of bacteria, including those that cause infections in the digestive system, reproductive system, and skin.

Flagyl belongs to a class of drugs called nitroimidazoles and works by disrupting the DNA of the bacteria or parasite, preventing it from replicating and causing further infection. It is a bactericidal antibiotic, meaning that it kills the bacteria rather than just inhibiting its growth. This makes it a very effective treatment for a wide range of infections.

Indications

Flagyl is primarily used to treat infections caused by anaerobic bacteria, meaning bacteria that can survive without oxygen. These types of bacteria are often found in areas of the body that have low oxygen levels, such as the digestive tract, reproductive organs, and deep wounds. Flagyl is commonly prescribed for the following conditions:

1. Bacterial Vaginosis: This is a common vaginal infection caused by an overgrowth of bacteria. Flagyl is the first-line treatment for bacterial vaginosis, with a success rate of over 90%.

2. Trichomoniasis: This is a sexually transmitted infection caused by a parasite. Flagyl is the drug of choice for treating trichomoniasis, with a cure rate of over 95%.

3. Intra-abdominal Infections: These are infections that occur inside the abdominal cavity, such as peritonitis, which is inflammation of the abdominal lining. Flagyl is used in combination with other antibiotics to treat these infections.

4.   Pseudomembranous Colitis: This is an infection of the colon caused by an overgrowth of the bacteria Clostridium difficile. Flagyl is often used to treat this condition, along with other antibiotics.

5.   Helicobacter pylori Infection: This is a bacterial infection that can cause stomach ulcers. Flagyl is used along with other antibiotics to eradicate the bacteria and treat the ulcer.

6. Skin and Soft Tissue Infections: Flagyl can be used to treat certain skin and soft tissue infections caused by anaerobic bacteria, such as cellulitis, abscesses, and infected wounds.

7. Bone and Joint Infections: Flagyl may be used in combination with other antibiotics to treat bone and joint infections, especially those caused by anaerobic bacteria.

8. Central Nervous System Infections: Flagyl is sometimes used in combination with other antibiotics to treat central nervous system infections, such as brain abscesses, meningitis, and spinal cord abscesses.

Flagyl is also used off-label for treating other infections, such as dental and respiratory infections, as well as certain types of diarrhea, including those caused by specific bacteria such as Clostridium difficile.

Chapter 2

Dosage and Administration

Flagyl is available in a variety of forms, including tablets, capsules, and injectable solutions. The dosage and duration of treatment will depend on the type and severity of the infection. It is important to follow the instructions provided by your doctor or on the medication label.

For bacterial vaginosis and trichomoniasis, a single dose

of 2 grams is usually prescribed, or a course of 500 mg taken twice daily for 7 days. In general, Flagyl is taken orally, with or without food, but it can also be administered intravenously in severe cases.

For other infections, the usual dose is 500 mg taken twice daily for 7-10 days. In some cases, a higher dosage may be prescribed, such as 750 mg taken 3 times daily for 7 days.

Possible Side Effects

As with any medication, Flagyl comes with a risk of side effects. The most common side effects include nausea, vomiting, diarrhea, abdominal pain, and loss of appetite. These side effects are usually mild and resolve on their own, but if they persist or become severe, it is important to speak to your doctor.

Some people may also experience a metallic taste in their mouth, which can be reduced by sucking on hard candy or chewing gum. In rare cases, more serious side effects can occur, such as allergic reactions, seizures, and nerve damage. If you experience any of these symptoms, seek immediate

We will discuss the potential side effects of Flagyl in details.

1. Gastrointestinal Distress

One of the most common side effects experienced by patients taking Flagyl is gastrointestinal distress. This can include symptoms such as nausea, vomiting, stomach pain, and diarrhea. These symptoms can be mild and often resolve on their own, but they can also be severe and may require medical attention. It is important to stay hydrated if experiencing severe diarrhea or vomiting while taking Flagyl.

2. Headaches and Dizziness

Some patients may also experience headaches or dizziness while taking Flagyl.

These symptoms are usually mild and can be managed with over-the-counter pain relievers. However, if they persist or become severe, patients should consult their healthcare provider.

3. Changes in Taste

Another common side effect of Flagyl is changes in taste. Patients may experience a metallic or bitter taste in their mouth while taking this medication. This can alter the taste of food and beverages and can be quite unpleasant.

While this side effect usually resolves once treatment is completed, some patients may continue to experience it for several weeks.

4. Allergic Reactions

Serious allergic reactions to Flagyl are rare, but they can occur. Symptoms of an allergic reaction may include hives, difficulty breathing, and swelling of the face, lips, tongue, or throat. If experiencing any of these symptoms, patients should seek medical attention immediately.

5. Nerve Damage

In rare cases, Flagyl can cause nerve damage, known as peripheral neuropathy. This is more likely to occur in patients who have a history of nerve damage or in those who take this medication for an extended period of time. Symptoms of peripheral neuropathy may include numbness, tingling, or weakness in the hands or feet. If experiencing these symptoms, patients should consult their healthcare provider.

6. Liver Damage

Flagyl can also cause liver damage in some patients. This is more likely to happen in those who have a history of liver disease or who take this medication for an extended period of time. Symptoms of liver damage may include yellowing of the skin or eyes (jaundice), dark urine, fatigue, or abdominal pain. Patients who experience these symptoms should seek medical attention immediately.

7. Blood Disorders

Rarely, Flagyl can cause changes in blood cells, leading to blood disorders such as anemia or a decrease in white blood cells. This can increase the risk of infections and can cause symptoms such as weakness, paleness, or unusual bleeding or bruising. Patients should seek medical attention if they experience any of these symptoms while taking this medication.

8. Nausea and Headaches

Some patients may experience more serious side effects such as seizures, difficulty speaking or controlling movements, or confusion. These are rare but potentially serious side effects that require immediate medical attention.

9. Interactions with Other Medications

Flagyl can interact with other medications, especially blood thinners and medications that treat psychiatric disorders. Patients should inform their healthcare provider of all medications they are taking before starting Flagyl.

10. Effects on Fertility

Some studies have shown that Flagyl can cause temporary infertility in men. It is important for patients to discuss any concerns about fertility with their healthcare provider before starting this medication.

11. Pregnancy and Breastfeeding

Flagyl is generally considered safe to use during pregnancy, but patients should discuss the potential risks with their healthcare provider. This medication can also pass into breast milk, so patients should consult their healthcare provider before taking Flagyl while breastfeeding.

Chapter 3

Precautions and Interactions

Flagyl should not be taken by people who are allergic to metronidazole or any other nitroimidazole antibiotics. It is also not recommended for pregnant or breastfeeding women, as it may pass into breast milk and harm the baby. It is important to inform your doctor of any other medications you are taking, as Flagyl may interact with other drugs, such as blood thinners, anticonvulsants, and certain antidepressants.

While taking Flagyl, it is important to avoid consuming alcohol, as it can lead to severe nausea, vomiting, and abdominal pain. It is also advised to avoid sexual intercourse during treatment for trichomoniasis and bacterial vaginosis, as this can spread the infection to your partner or cause reinfection.

In rare cases, long-term use of Flagyl may result in a condition called peripheral neuropathy, which causes numbness, tingling, and pain in the hands and feet. This usually resolves once the medication is stopped, but it is important to report any symptoms to your doctor.

Chapter 4

Conclusion

Flagyl is a powerful and effective antibiotic that has been in use for over 60 years. It is used to treat a wide range of infections caused by bacteria and parasites, and it has a high success rate. However, as with any medication, there are certain precautions to be taken and potential side effects to be aware of.

It is important to always follow your doctor's instructions and take the medication as prescribed. If you experience any side effects or have concerns about the medication, do not hesitate to speak to your doctor. With proper use and monitoring, Flagyl can help to treat and prevent various infections, improving the health and well-being of millions of people worldwide.

While Flagyl can effectively treat bacterial infections, it is important to be aware of its potential side effects. Patients should inform their healthcare provider if they experience any of these side effects, and seek medical attention if they have any concerns. It is also important to follow the prescribed dosage and complete the full course of treatment to ensure the infection is fully cleared and to minimize the risk of developing antibiotic resistance.

THE END

Made in United States
Troutdale, OR
02/25/2024

17958641R00020